I0447705

E-Cigarettes: 'Re-inventing smoking'

Creating a new generation of smokers

by

Karl A. Cox, PhD

The purpose of this book

It is apparent simply from observation that electronic cigarettes are becoming the new tobacco in the Westernised world. High streets in most towns now have one or more dedicated e-cigarette store. Traditional tobacconists are now promoting electronic cigarettes in order to compete. All supermarkets that sell cigarettes now have a big and open-to-see electronic cigarettes range and promote

e-cigarettes *in big letters. Petrol stations place e-cigarettes on their counters right beside children's football cards at their point of sales. Go look. These are the consequence of and at the same time promoter of three phenomena we are now seeing in action:*

1. *The promotion that an electronic cigarette is harmless to the person vaping it and to the person inhaling the secondhand vapour.*
2. *As a consequence of 1 above, that vaping is acceptable social behaviour and should be encouraged.*
3. *Again as a consequence, that the inhaling of anything into the lungs containing a toxic content is good.*

Phenomenon 1 is proven false – e-cigarettes are harmful; they contain toxins that cause cancer. The accepted science shows this. This book will describe the contents found in e-cigarettes and their effect. E-cigarettes are addictive because the vast majority are nicotine delivery devices... just like tobacco cigarettes. So those who vape are trapped and are poisoning themselves. More of this later but to prove the point right now. In a published study in the Journal of Respiratory Research, *scientists at the University of Manchester found that e-cigarette vapour causes inflammation on the lungs similar to that of tobacco smoke[1]. The researchers found inflammatory markers in e-cigarette vapour have a similar effect to those produced by tobacco smoking which cause chronic obstructive pulmonary disease (COPD). This inflammation is caused by e-cigarette vapour whose contents also contain many carcinogens, such as "saturated aldehyde propanol, the carcinogens 2, 3-benzofuran and allylthiourea and the respiratory toxin styrene ...[and] acrolein in the vapour extract but not the e-liquid itself... Acrolein is also a constituent of tobacco smoke."[2]*

Phenomenon 2 is proven false because Phenomenon 1 is false. Also, vaping as acceptable is illusion put forth by the manufacturers of these products in order to sell more products. Their motivation is money. They do not care about the health effects of vaping. This is proven simply through observation of how Big Tobacco behaved in order to sell tobacco. They lied in order to make money and they knew it. Now the owners of electronic cigarette companies are predominantly the very same Big Tobacco companies who lied for decades about the addictiveness of and toxins in tobacco cigarettes[3].

Phenomenon 3, that to inhale a substance containing toxins into one's lungs is somehow good, is baffling. This premise cannot make sense whichever way you look at it. It is false. To inhale nicotine and carcinogens, heavy metals and toxins into one's lungs, yet be told this is fine, healthy and normal, as I said, is baffling. Lungs are designed to inhale air, from which energy is transferred into the blood to bring life and to restore and heal, not to poison.

One side effect of the promotion of acceptance of electronic cigarettes is that the children and youth who try e-cigarettes are more likely to turn to tobacco cigarettes later. In the United States of America, a study published in the journal Pediatrics *shows that teenagers who vaped e-cigarettes were* six *times more likely to take up smoking tobacco cigarettes.[4]*

The survey reported in Pediatrics *found that 24 per cent of teenagers (mean age 17) had tried electronic cigarettes. An earlier survey conducted by the Centers for Disease Control and Prevention (CDC) in the United States highlights that e-cigarette use tripled among school children from 2011 to 2014[5]. The* Pediatrics *study indicates that the upward trend is continuing: more and more school children are taking to electronic cigarettes. The use of e-cigarettes is skyrocketing in the US and around the world among children and teenagers – e-cigarettes are now mostly owned by tobacco companies: a new generation of smokers is being created.*

Is this acceptable behavior that should be promoted? Of course not, but this is what is happening. We've seen this all before with tobacco cigarettes where false advertised such as the notorious case of actors playing doctors who made claims that smoking not only is harmless but in fact beneficial. A result of this is millions of lives ruined through disease and death, and the tobacco industry becoming massively rich as a consequence.

Will we permit history to repeat itself and allow e-cigarettes into the hands of children and teenagers or even adults without a really honest appraisal? It seems to be the case that governments have wised up enough to ban the sale of e-cigarettes to minors. There's enough distrust of the tobacco industry to recognize this. The academic publishing world has finally woken up also to the idea that tobacco industry-funded studies might be somewhat biased towards promoting the benefits of their own products by identifying fewer negative health effects than there are. As an example, in March 2014, the European Journal of Public Health announced it would no longer publish tobacco industry-supported research:

"The European Journal of Public Health will no longer consider for publication any study that is partly or wholly funded by the tobacco industry. In doing so, it falls into line with the long-standing policy of journals such as Tobacco Control, PLoS Medicine, PLoS One, PLoS Biology and the Journal of Health Psychology, joined in October 2013 by the BMJ, Heart, Thorax and BMJ Open."[6] It is still astonishing to many that the leading medical and health publications such as the British Medical Journal[7] took so long to announce they would no longer accept any tobacco industry funded research. Why was this? Corporations have a history – in many diverse fields – in placing their people or sympathisers to their cause on the editorial boards of scientific journals. So when a paper with negative findings about their product comes in, they work to ensure it doesn't get published and when something biased in favour of a toxic product is submitted for publication, the pro-industry editor works to promote the paper for publication, finding reviewers with the same belief in order to ensure a seemingly fair and honest peer-review process, which of course it is not.

So where do the research journals stand in regard to electronic cigarettes? Are they equally as suspicious of e-cigarette promotion as they are of tobacco? Or has the wool been pulled over their eyes again, and over the eyes of government and and over the eyes of the public?

Introduction

Electronic cigarettes are devices that have become popular in many countries as tobacco cigarette substitutes or smoking cessation devices. E-cigarettes mimic smoking in that a user inhales a vapour rather than smoke. Their uptake in many countries has been dramatic. It was reported that the UK Office for National Statistics (ONS) estimated in February 2016 there were 2.2 million e-cigarette users, 4 per cent of the population[8]. This number increased by 800,000 within two years and is short of today's actual number of at least 2.8 million e-cigarettes users in the UK, as published by Public Health England in July 2016[9]. As of time of writing (September 2016), this figure could already be at the 3 million mark. E-cigarettes have become a big industry.

For teenagers and children in the Western world, "vaping" is replacing tobacco cigarettes as the choice for smoking. This is ensuring a new generation of smokers for the producers of electronic cigarettes. The main producers of e-cigarettes are the Big Tobacco companies. The way in which electronic cigarettes are marketed reflects the worst of tobacco advertising of years gone by: sexual imagery and targeting children.

Are electronic cigarettes harmless and do they really help you quit?

The independent scientific research and government research is now showing that:

1) Electronic cigarettes do not help smokers quit the habit – in most cases, those using electronic cigarettes continue to smoke and in the case of those who do quit tobacco, they continue to vape.
2) Electronic cigarettes contain many carcinogenic and toxic substances – they are not harmless at all.

This book's goal is to bring awareness of the evidence of the danger of electronic cigarettes to governments, to doctors, to smokers who want to quit and have explored e-cigarettes as a cessation device, and to those who are considering vaping as a hobby, especially the youth who are turning to e-cigarettes at an alarming rate. I want to make it clear here that smoking in any of its forms is not going to help anyone. Tobacco kills six million people a year – a true pandemic that is as good as ignored by governments globally. The tobacco industry needs to be put out of existence. The harm its products cause is truly shocking. So please don't think for a second this book recommends smokers should not quit. All I am saying here is that electronic cigarettes are wolves in sheeps' clothing. They are marketed as harmless but in actual fact they are addictive and full of dangerous toxins, chemicals and poisons. There are much better ways to quit smoking than turning to e-cigarettes. These will be explored later and sources of advice and help recommended. What I am saying is that electronic cigarettes are part of the problem, not the solution; that e-cigarettes have been painted as a saviour, contrary to much of the scientific evidence thus far; that the industry promoting electronic cigarettes is the tobacco industry and that is an industry we simply cannot trust.

How e-cigarettes work

An e-cigarette is a smokeless cigarette that contains no tobacco and is not lit with a flame nor burns as a flame. It is a device that heats, via a battery on to an 'atomiser', a cocktail of liquid chemicals, often including nicotine, that is converted into a vapour. This vapour is then inhaled, imitating smoking.

The first electronic cigarettes looked like tobacco cigarettes and had a light at the end that illuminated when a user inhaled. More recently, e-cigarettes look more like fountain pens, or hookah pens. They have a larger refillable reservoir so you can get more puffs than before, and so can reuse the e-cigarette rather than throw it away.

Nicotine hit

The first vape is similar in concept to the first cigarette. Nicotine hits the brain with waves of 'feel-goodness' but as with tobacco smoke, the body is hit at the same time with a multitude of chemicals and heavy metals. Nicotine imitates the neurotransmitter *acetylcholine*. This transmitter goes on to trigger the release of dopamine, which activates 'reward' pathways in the brain, the same as cocaine does, meaning the smoker or the vaper gets a feel good feeling and the desire to get that feeling again – the highly addictive property of nicotine, the craving for the next vape or smoke. But coupled with this feel-good inducer, is the opposite effect of depression and poisons. Heavy metals are known to cause a feeling of depression. So to alleviate this feeling 'down', the smoker, or the vaper, takes another puff to get that nicotine rush, that makes everything feel wonderful again. But only for a short period of time until the depressing heavy metals and other toxins make the vaper's body and mind feel low. And then it is time for that nicotine hit again. And so it goes on. And the smoker and the vaper are addicted from the first inhalation.

Many e-cigarette users can be observed taking two inhalations in close succession, one immediately after the other, in situations where there is no pressure to put the e-cigarette away, such as upon entering a building or getting on the bus. Why is this the case? Could a plausible answer be the following? That because there is less nicotine in an e-cigarette inhalation than in tobacco, this may be why e-cigarette users who were or still are tobacco users need to take two inhalations in rapid succession of the e-cigarette vapour to get the level of nicotine to amounts found in a single tobacco inhalation so that the dopamine can be released at levels they are used to and need? They are still addicted to the level of nicotine in tobacco cigarettes and this will explain why ex-smokers are turning to e-cigarettes: they have not conquered their nicotine addiction. And it explains why dual users (those using both tobacco and e-cigarettes) don't give up on tobacco – they may not be getting enough nicotine from e-cigarettes to be able to give up the tobacco. This also explains why e-cigarette users may take up tobacco smoking or return to tobacco smoking if they are ex-tobacco users: they have not been able to quit their nicotine addiction. BUT, these individuals may have been misled into thinking that e-cigarettes are harmless compared to tobacco through the marketing and advertising campaigns of both the industry, governments and anti-smoking non-governmental organisations or charities. It is also the case, as recognized with tobacco smoking that the longer a person has smoked, the less the nicotine will have a feel good effect. This is because the body has accumulated poisons, toxins and heavy metals from the cigarette that are having a larger negative effect and as the brain becomes so used to nicotine it no longer reacts with the same elation as before. So smokers smoke more as they get older. The same holds true for e-cigarette users because they are taking in nicotine and many of the poisons, toxins and heavy metals found in tobacco. Not all the poisons are there but many still are. Tar is not found in electronic cigarettes and this is because e-cigarettes do not burn tobacco.

Smokers who take to e-cigarettes are certainly aware that e-cigarettes are at least as harmful to health as tobacco. A survey conducted as part of the 'Smoking Toolkit Study' by University College London found this to be the case as seen in the following graph:

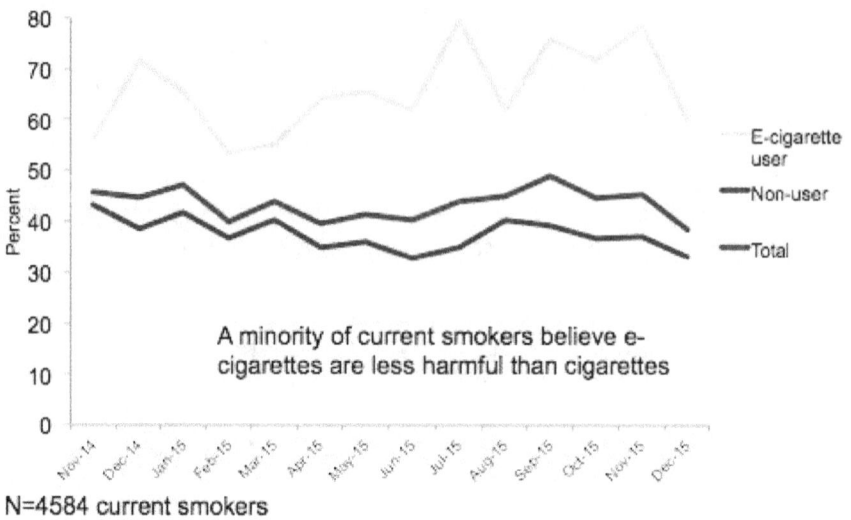

N=4584 current smokers

Graph taken from: http://www.smokinginengland.info/latest-statistics/

The graph states, and I quote, "A minority of current [tobacco] smokers believe e-cigarettes are less harmful than cigarettes." Repeat: only a minority of smokers believes e-cigarettes are *less* harmful than tobacco. Why are we led to believe by some scientists, doctors and governments that e-cigarettes are not harmful?

Why do people smoke?

A wise man once said, "You can't be intelligent and smoke at the same time!" So why do people start smoking and why are electronic cigarettes becoming the smoking fashion?

Much of the reason is peer pressure or being raised in a family of smokers or being rebellious and feeling this is somehow sexy. Indeed, the marketing of e-cigarettes has played on this significantly.

How are electronic cigarettes marketed?

If we turn the clock back to the 1970s we see advertisements showing sophisticated women and rugged men reaching for a tobacco cigarette to light up. The public image of smoking, for men at least, was the Marlboro man.

The marketing approach of today is no different to tobacco advertising. E-cigarettes are promoted by movie stars, attractive young men and and women, with an air of rebelliousness, and with sexually provocative advertisements.

E-cigarette companies, that is, for the most part, tobacco companies, are spending millions in marketing campaigns from billboard posters, to television adverts.

Though figures have varied, the UK now boasts at least 2.8 million e-cigarette smokers (as of July 2016) and this figure may be much more. It will also rise as teen and 20-something audiences are targeted through sexually explicit advertisements. One advertisement implied an e-cigarette experience was an explicit sex act[10] and one, British American Tobacco, promoted e-cigarettes to young children in a computer game advertisement[11].

Vapestick, a UK e-cigarette company, advertised via a 'search for a Style Icon'. You can see immediately that we are now in the realm of the 'Marlboro Man', that rugged, cool individual who is the personification of the smoker, so that you feel something like James Bond just because you smoke. Vapestick's search for its own Marlboro Man or Woman is no different: it is all and only about making money for them. Marlboro Man died in 2014 of a smoking related disease and was the 5th actor in such as role to die because of smoking[12].

The British Medical Journal has noted that e-cigarette marketing seems to be tobacco marketing reinvented, with marketing expenditure on e-cigarettes on the increase from £1 million in 2010 to £13 million in 2011. In 2013, British American Tobacco promoted its Vype e-cigarette in the UK, spending £3.6 million in only two months[13]. Indeed, the ethics of marketing e-cigarettes in the UK is now under investigation; without knowing the true health effects of these products, marketing them is viewed as a return to the age of tobacco[14].

Public Health England (PHE), the UK non-Governmental Agency advising the government on health matters and policy, reports:

"The e-cigarette market is estimated to be worth £91.3 million a year. It increased by 340% in 2013 to reach £193 million, and is expected to be worth £340 million by 2015." (p4)[15].

The PHE reports on Big Tobacco's activity in e-cigarettes:

- British American Tobacco acquired CN Creative (maker of e-cigarette Intellicig) in 2012 and launched the Vype e-cigarette.
- Imperial Tobacco formed the wholly-owned subsidiary Fontem Ventures to develop 'e-vapour cigarettes'.
- Lorillard (in the US) acquired Blu in 2012 for £90 million and Skycig for £30 million in 2013.
- Altria (owner of Philip Morris) launched its own e-cig, MarkTen, in 2013 and paid £66 million for Green Smoke Inc in 2014.

Marketing goes beyond solely the electronic cigarette. We now have a host of variations and new products supporting 'vaping' and 'vapers' on the market:

- There are now a huge variety of weird flavours to try[16]. Are these flavours, such as bubblegum aimed at the younger generation, that is, school children?
- You can now hook your mobile phone, via Bluetooth, to an e-cigarette, meaning you can take calls or play music whilst vaping, without touching your mobile phone[17].
- Blu ECigs launched a smart e-cigarette detector to link you with someone within fifty feet also using the same e-cigarette brand to connect you together on Facebook and Twitter.[18] One goal of this could be to create a community of vapers where vaping is viewed as the norm, and as such those vaping are less likely to quit.
- E-cigarettes now have apps running from iPhones to tell the smoker how much money they saved from using the e-cigarette compared to tobacco, the number of puffs taken and whether there is possibly less harm caused by the e-cigarette compared to tobacco.[19] How this app can say you are causing less harm is a mystery when e-cigarette producers are not open about their ingredients.

The Public Health England report states that more money is going into marketing:

"Skycig also recently announced its investment in a £20 million marketing campaign including television advertising and public relations (PR) companies have now been appointed to reposition Skycig as 'a positive lifestyle choice for smokers'. Marketing strategies will focus 'on passion points stretching from sport to fashion' and music. Most competitor companies have also hired advertising and PR agencies to promote expensive 'above-the-line' marketing campaigns."

Growing market for electronic cigarettes

It is easy to see why the tobacco industry has taken a strong interest in the electronic-cigarette market. In 2014, the UK had over 2.1 million e-cigarette users[20]. This is rapidly increasing in number with last estimates of 2.8 million in July 2016, probably haven risen already to 3 million or more by the time you read this book. This is a multi-million dollar business. In the United States of America, the market size is over $1 billion annually, and growing rapidly.

Wells Fargo estimates that sales margins for e-cigarettes may grow to $10 billion by 2017, surpassing tobacco cigarette sales margins, predicting that Big Tobacco could own 75% of the e-cigarette profit pool in 10 years[21].

History of the e-cigarette

The e-cigarette was invented by Herbert A. Gilbert in 1963 but the product did not go commercial. The e-cigarette became a commercial product in 2003 through the efforts of a Chinese pharmacist called Hon Lik. The e-cigarette went on sale in May 2004 in China and the company Hon Lik worked for re-named itself from Golden Dragon Holdings to Ruyan (literally meaning "resembling smoking") so it could export the product from 2005.

Big Tobacco has moved into the e-cigarette market through acquisition and manufacturing their own products. For example, Lorriard acquired Blu, an e-cigarette company. British American Tobacco recently launched its own e-cigarette range called Vype. Imperial Tobacco acquired the intellectual property owned by Hon Lik through Dragonite for $US 75 million.[22]

Do e-cigarettes help smokers quit?

There is growing evidence that e-cigarettes do not help smokers quit, do contain harmful substances, are being marketed like tobacco products were and that children are turning to e-cigarettes instead of tobacco.[23]

According to one expert, Dr Matthew Mintz, "e-cigarettes were designed to be tobacco cigarette replacement products, not smoking cessation aides. It is also possible that smokers will use e-cigarettes in place of SOME of their tobacco cigarettes. Although this does decrease exposure to known dangerous products, e-cigarettes might therefore actually prolong tobacco cigarette smoking."[24]

A key ingredient for most e-cigarettes is nicotine. The American government agency, Drug Abuse, states this about nicotine:

"Most smokers use tobacco regularly because they are addicted to nicotine. Addiction is characterized by compulsive drug seeking and abuse, even in the face of negative health consequences. It is well documented that most smokers identify tobacco use as harmful and express a desire to reduce or stop using it, and nearly 35 million of them want to quit each year. Unfortunately, more than 85 percent of those who try to quit on their own relapse, most within a week.

"Research has shown how nicotine acts on the brain to produce a number of effects. Of primary importance to its addictive nature are findings that nicotine activates reward pathways—the brain circuitry that regulates feelings of pleasure. A key brain chemical involved in mediating the desire to consume drugs is the neurotransmitter dopamine, and research has shown that nicotine increases levels of dopamine in the reward circuits. This reaction is similar to that seen with other drugs of abuse and is thought to underlie the pleasurable sensations experienced by many smokers. For many tobacco users, long-term brain changes induced by continued nicotine exposure result in addiction."[25]

Electronic cigarettes typically contain nicotine. This means that electronic cigarettes are addiction-forming devices. How can this help people quit? It may be the case that those who turn to e-cigarettes to help them quit are *less likely* to quit. One study published in the *American Journal of Public Health* found:

"Smokers who used e-cigarettes were 49 percent less likely to decrease cigarette use and 59 percent less likely to quit smoking compared to smokers who never used e-cigarettes."[26]

This is corroborated by a move in the City of Philadelphia to ban e-cigarettes from public places amid concerns that "a new study shows smokers who use them aren't more likely to quit or reduce cigarette use after a year. And there's some concern that e-cigarettes may lead young people to try other tobacco products."[27]

The new study referred to was reported in *Nature*[28]. The actual study itself, is published in *JAMA Internal Medicine*[29]. The year-long study reports that there was no difference between e-cigarette user and cigarette user quitting rates. In other words, smoking e-cigarettes made it no easier to quit than if smoking tobacco cigarettes. Given that the primary ingredient in e-cigarettes is nicotine, a most highly addictive substance, this should come as no surprise.

Dramatic increase in numbers of children trying e-cigarettes

The City of Philadelphia's move to ban e-cigarettes in public places can be understood if we look at the alarming up-take of e-cigarettes by children and youths.

In August 2014, the US Government Agency, Centers for Disease Control and Prevention (CDC) announced that in 2013, more than a quarter of a million youth in the United States who had never tried a tobacco cigarette tried an electronic cigarette; this number was three times higher than in 2011.[30]

Since then, The CDC has been reported that the number of middle and high school students trying or using an e-cigarette has tripled from 2013 to 2014 to 2 million[31].

In the UK, it was reported by the Welsh Government that children in Wales are three times as likely to try e-cigarettes than tobacco.[32] This has led to the Welsh Government outlawing vaping in enclosed public spaces and at work[33]. In a study published in *Pediatrics* on 15 December 2014, a comparison was made of tobacco uptake against e-cigarette uptake in the US among adolescents. The findings show that adolescents who are considered to have a reduced risk of trying tobacco because of their demographic are taking to e-cigarettes instead.[34] What the evidence is now showing is that children are the targets of this product and it is the reason why we have seen such an enormous increase in marketing.

This danger, the risk of creating a new generation of "smokers" held in the clutches of Big Tobacco is recognized in the US. The Washington Post calls for a ban on sales and advertising of e-cigarettes to under 18 year-olds. Robert McCartney writes if people want to 'vape' that is up to them "But that doesn't mean the public should allow Big Tobacco to use its billions to build a new mass market for a consumer product scientifically proved to be very addictive."[35] This, in response to a report by Senator Richard Durbin and fellow Senators and Representatives into how e-cigarette manufacturers are deliberately targeting youth and young generations to hook them into a lifetime dependency on e-cigarettes.[36]

Are electronic cigarettes harmful to health?

The World Health Organisation (WHO) is taking action to classify e-cigarettes as a health threat[37]. The European Union is in the process of deciding what to do about e-cigarettes. Its parliamentary committee has stated it will consider all e-cigarettes as pharmaceutical products and hence that they can only be sold like other smoking cessation aids such as patches.[38] The US Government is considering this legislative move also.

Liquid poison

Nicotine in liquid form, which is used in electronic cigarettes, is a poison. This is well documented. Chemists know that nicotine, in its liquid form, is highly toxic. It is more toxic than arsenic and strychnine.[39] The nicotine liquid used in e-cigarettes can kill, even when in contact with the skin. This is especially a risk for children but also for household pets. The CDC reports an increase in calls to poison centres involving e-cigarette nicotine liquids from 1 per month in September 2010 to 215 in the month on February 2014[40].

The New York Times ran an article on 23rd March 2014 entitled *Selling a Poison by the Barrel: Liquid Nicotine for E-Cigarettes*, in which it states it is not a matter of if a child will be poisoned and die but a matter of when.[41] Sadly, it has happened – a toddler lost his life after ingesting the nicotine liquid.[42] Any further debate on the health risk of the liquid nicotine is now lame – it is a killer.

What is in the e-cigarette liquid and vapour?

"We do not yet know the harm that e-cigarettes can cause to adults, let alone to children, but we do know they are not risk free," Professor Dame Sally Davies, England's chief medical officer, said. "E-cigarettes can produce toxic chemicals and the amount of nicotine and other chemical constituents and contaminants, including vaporised flavourings, varies between products - meaning they could be extremely damaging to young people's health."[43]

The American Agency, the Foods and Drugs Administration, though not actively investigated e-cigarettes, is actively collating individual accounts of health effects of e-cigarettes and to date they write that the following list led to hospitalization in some cases:
- "pneumonia,
- congestive heart failure,
- disorientation,
- seizure,
- hypotension, and
- other health problems."[44]

In a report in a French Magazine, *60 Millions Consommateurs* (60 Million Consumers) – "which reports the findings of the National Consumers' Institute - said it tested ten different rechargeable and disposable models [of e-cigarettes] for carcinogenic and toxic properties. Editor Thomas Laurenceau wrote: 'We detected a significant quantity of carcinogenic molecules in the vapour of these cigarettes which have thus far gone undetected. In three models out of ten the levels of the carcinogenic compound formaldehyde come close to those of a conventional cigarette. The highly toxic molecule acrolein was also detected in the vapours of e-cigarettes, sometimes at levels even higher than in traditional cigarettes.'"[45]

There is evidence that e-cigarettes are putting lungs under significant stress from the first.[46] "We found an immediate rise in airway resistance in our group of participants, which suggests e-cigarettes can cause immediate harm after smoking the device," Professor Christina Gratziou, Chair of the European Respiratory Society Tobacco Control Committee reported. The article comments on the confusion about the danger of e-cigarettes in comparison to tobacco: "We do not yet know whether unapproved nicotine delivery products, such as e-cigarettes, are safer than normal cigarettes, despite marketing claims that they are less harmful."

Professor Bertrand Dautzenberg states, "E-cigarettes are toxic, addictive and not for young people."[47] In an article posted in May 2014, Dr Mercola states:

"The highly toxic liquid in e-cigarettes is responsible for a surge of child poisonings; just one teaspoon may be enough to kill your child. E-cigarettes contain toxic agents manufacturers are reluctant to disclose, such as lead, benzene, toluene, and formaldehyde."[48]

Secondhand vapour

Also, it is not just the vaper who is at risk; just as there is secondhand smoking, there is secondhand vaping:

"If you are around somebody who is using e-cigarettes, you are breathing an aerosol of exhaled nicotine, ultra-fine particles, volatile organic compounds, and other toxins," states Dr. Stanton Glantz, Director for the Center for Tobacco Control Research and Education at the University of California, San Francisco[49].

A study conducted by the Fraunhofer Institute in Germany found that there are enough ultrafine particles exhaled from an e-cigarette to show passive vaping is occurring.[50]

Public Health England (PHE), an allegedly independent body, provides advice to government on policy. In its July 2016 published advice, PHE does not accept there is evidence of secondhand vaping and that the risk is negligent. In the same document, it states:

"while it is preferable for young people neither to smoke nor to vape, when assessing the risks policies should give priority to supporting young people not to smoke."[51]

What exactly does this imply? That given the choice between smoking and vaping, we should encourage children to vape? But this is entirely the wrong advice, and is entirely stupid on the part of Public Health England. One would think they want children to get sick and have a life of addiction to e-cigarettes and then tobacco. Surely any sane person would advise their children or any child or youth, no, do not try either, both are toxic, both are addictive and both are dangerous? Perhaps I am mistakenly presuming PHE as sane as the rest of us? Yes, PHE does says it prefers young people not to smoke or vape; well, then make the most of that and call for a ban on both. Don't state one thing then wriggle out of it in the next breath for that is disgraceful.

Compare Public Health England to the United States of America:

On 25th August 2014, the American Heart Association published a review and policy statement of e-cigarettes. One of the most important points they make is this:

"*Proponents of e-cigarettes maintain that these products emulate smoking behavior without exposing the user to the toxic smoke constituents of conventional cigarettes that are deleterious to health, so there would be a public health benefit if individual smokers completely switched or substantially reduced their cigarette smoking habit. However, the use of e-cigarettes could be a problem at the population level. For instance, e-cigarettes could fuel and promote nicotine addiction, especially in children, and their acceptance has the potential to renormalize smoking behavior. E-cigarette use could also potentially serve as a gateway to other drugs and harmful substances.*"[52]

In the US, and to some extent in the UK, it is prohibited to smoke in public places such as restaurants or the office. The US calls these 'smoke-free air laws' that are vital to protecting air quality. The UK's PHE does not think this is important. The American Heart Association (AHA) consider "*unregulated e-cigarette use has the potential to recreate a social norm around tobacco product use in public places, unraveling decades of work on comprehensive smoke-free air laws... E-cigarette companies are marketing their products to be used in all the places where smoking is banned, including bars, restaurants, hotels, offices, and airplanes.*" [Ref: American Heart Association policy statement 24 August 2014.] The World Health Organisation agrees with the AHA in its declaration that e-cigarettes should be banned indoors.[53]

The AHA policy statement also indicates that nicotine addiction is just as strong with e-cigarettes as with tobacco because some, but not all, e-cigarettes allow for amounts of nicotine to be vaped similar to a tobacco cigarette. This nicotine is taken into the lungs and absorbed as a vapour, rather than smoke. Secondhand vapers may not receive the same kind of smoke that they would from tobacco but "*non-smokers are exposed to some nicotine, and the regular use of e-cigarettes has the potential to substantially contaminate the environment with nicotine,*" [A. Bhatnagar *et al.* (2014) AHA Policy Statement, p.8].

In 2016, United States Food and Drugs Administration began regulation of e-cigarettes and places them in the same category as tobacco cigarettes.[54] This is in strong contrast to the UK Government that has gone the other way and state there is little to no evidence of harm. How can these two nations be poles apart? What is driving the agenda for the UK Government? The evidence coming from the US is clear.

Vaping during pregnancy?

Women should not turn to e-cigarettes as a safe option for smoking during pregnancy. An American study on the effects of e-cigarette vapour on pregnant mice, as reported in the *Evening Standard* states:

"The early findings, based on studies of mice, show that exposure to volatile chemicals from the devices [e-cigarettes] disrupts the activity of thousands of genes in the developing [baby's] brain.

"Analysis of the altered gene activity patterns indicated that they could lead to reductions in learning, memory and co-ordination, and increases in hyperactive behaviour.

"These are just the sort of neurological effects seen in children whose mothers smoked during pregnancy and who are known to be at risk of attention deficit hyperactivity disorder (ADHD) and learning difficulties."[55]

This news, reported globally, followed a press release by the American Association for the Advancement of Science held on 11th February 2016 at their annual meeting in Washington, DC.[56]

Proof of carcinogens

In a published study conducted in Japan, it was found that one electronic cigarette brand, whose name was undisclosed, contained **10 times** the level of formaldehyde found in some tobacco cigarettes.

As reported in *The Guardian* newspaper on November 28th 2014[57]:

"Researchers at Japan's National Institute for Public Health said they had found two carcinogens - formaldehyde and acetaldehyde – in vapour produced by several types of e-cigarettes during a study commissioned by the country's health ministry.

"One brand of e-cigarette produced 10 times more formaldehyde – a substance used in embalming that has also been linked to sick building syndrome – than a regular cigarette, said Naoki Kunugita, who led the research.

"Especially when the wire (which vapourises the liquid) gets overheated, higher amounts of those harmful substances seemed to be produced... We need to be aware that some makers are selling such products for dual use (with tobacco) or as a gateway for young people [to start smoking]."

Known chemicals and toxins in e-cigarettes

The following table lists the chemicals and toxins found in electronic cigarettes that have been made public. There could be many more that are kept under "trade secrets" rules that we are not aware of yet, as was the case with tobacco.

Chemical/ Toxin	Can cause / Known for	Source
Nicotine	More addictive than heroin; deadly in liquid form as described above [1].	[1] Nicotine Addiction 101, http://whyquit.com/whyquit/LinksAAddiction.html
Nitric Oxide	Causes pulmonary inflammation 18, 29, 16% higher than baseline measures [1]	[1] D. Palazzolo (2013), Electronic Cigarettes and Vaping: A New Challenge in Clinical Medicine and Public Health. A Literature Review, *Front Public Health*. 2013; 1: 56, http://www.ncbi.nlm.nih.gov/pmc/articles/PMC3859972/
Acrolein	Presumed non-toxic but linked to lung cancer when smoked. Can be a byproduct of propylene when heated [1].	[1] Wikipedia, Acrolein, http://en.wikipedia.org/wiki/Acrolein#Health_risks
Lead	For children exposed to lead: "Behavior and learning problems; Lower IQ and Hyperactivity; Slowed growth; Hearing Problems; Anemia. In rare cases, ingestion of lead can cause seizures, coma and even death. For pregnant women, lead poisoning leads to smaller fetuses and premature births." [1] Level varies but found to be equivalent to or higher than in tobacco [2].	[1] United States Environmental Protection Agency, Learn about Lead, 21st April 2015, http://www2.epa.gov/lead/learn-about-lead#effects [2] Williams M, Villarreal A, Bozhilov K, Lin S, Talbot P. Metal and silicate particles including nanoparticles are present in electronic cigarette cartomizer fluid and aerosol. PLoS One (2013) 8:3.10.1371/journal.pone.0057987
Benzene	Damages bone marrow and causes anemia via red blood cell count reduction. This weakens the immune system and can lead to death [1]. The WHO says benzene exposure is a major public health concern and is listed by the WHO as a class 1 carcinogen (proven cause of cancer) [2].	[1] CDC, Facts about Benzene, 14th February 2013, http://www.bt.cdc.gov/agent/benzene/basics/facts.asp [2] World Health Organisation, Exposure to Benzene: A Major Public Health Concern, 2010, http://www.who.int/ipcs/features/benzene.pdf
Toluene	"A serious health concern is that toluene may have an effect on your brain. Toluene can cause headaches and sleepiness, and can impair your ability to think clearly. If you are exposed to a large amount of toluene in a short time because you deliberately sniff paint or glue [what about e-cigarettes?], you will first feel light-headed. If exposure continues, you can become dizzy, sleepy, or unconscious. You might even die. Toluene causes death by interfering with the way you breathe and the way your heart beats." [1] Toluene also can damage your kidneys and reproductive capabilities.	[1] Agency for Toxic Substances and Disease Registry, Public Health Statement for Toluene, September 2000, http://www.atsdr.cdc.gov/phs/phs.asp?id=159&tid=29
Formaldehyde	Cancer; leukemia; classified as a class 1	[1] National Cancer Institute,

	(proven) carcinogen by the WHO [1]. Formaldehyde was found in one study conducted in Japan to be 10 times higher than that found in tobacco cigarettes [2].	Formaldehyde and Cancer Risk, 10th June 2011, http://www.cancer.gov/cancertopics/factsheet/Risk/formaldehyde [2] The Guardian, Japan to investigate e-cigarette safety after formaldehyde findings, 28th November 2014, http://www.theguardian.com/society/2014/nov/28/japan-e-cigarette-safety
Ultrafine particles	Asthma, constricted arteries, heart attacks. Levels considered high enough in passive vaping to be a risk to health [1].	[1] Grana, R; Benowitz, N; Glantz, S. "Background Paper on E-cigarettes," Center for Tobacco Control Research and Education, University of California, San Francisco and WHO Collaborating Center on Tobacco Control. December 2013
Acetaldehyde	Causes cancer (class 1 carcinogen); damages DNA; "it may also cause drowsiness, delirium, hallucinations, and loss of intelligence. Exposure may also cause severe damage to the mouth, throat, and stomach; accumulation of fluid in the lungs, chronic respiratory disease, kidney and liver damage, throat irritation, dizziness, reddening, and swelling of the skin." [1] In a report by the New Zealand Government, it was found that Acetaldehyde was present but levels are unclear. Recommended to assess the exhaled amount. Some concern shown [2]	[1] Wikipedia, Acetaldehyde, http://en.wikipedia.org/wiki/Acetaldehyde#Dangers [2] M. Laugensen et al, How Safe Is An e-Cigarette? http://www.healthnz.co.nz/Portland2008ECIG.pdf
Cadmium	Highly toxic metal. "Inhaling cadmium-laden dust quickly leads to respiratory tract and kidney problems which can be fatal (often from renal failure). Ingestion of any significant amount of cadmium causes immediate poisoning and damage to the liver and the kidneys. Compounds containing cadmium are also carcinogenic." [1]	[1] Wikipedia, Cadmium, http://en.wikipedia.org/wiki/Cadmium_poisoning
Isoprene	Blood damage, spinal cord damage, reproductive organ failure, organ cancer [1]. Found in e-cigarettes but unclear what levels there are [2].	[1] R. Melnick, Isoprene, National Toxicology Program, Toxicity Report Series Number 31, United States Department of Health and Human Services, NIH Publication 94-3354 July 1994 http://ntp.niehs.nih.gov/ntp/htdocs/st_rpts/tox031.pdf [2] R. Grana et al, E-cigarettes: A Scientific Review, Circulation. May 13, 2014; 129(19): 1972–1986.
Nickel	Common effect is allergic reaction, respiratory problems such as bronchitis, lung failure; kidney problems [1]. 2 to 100 times higher than found in Marlboro cigarettes [2].	[1] Agency for Toxic Substances and Disease Registry, Public Health Statement for Nickel, August 2005, http://www.atsdr.cdc.gov/phs/phs.asp?id=243&tid=44#bookmark05

		[2] R. Grana et al, E-cigarettes: A Scientific Review, *Circulation*. May 13, 2014; 129(19): 1972–1986.
N-Nitrosonornicotine	Class 1 Carcinogen (WHO) [1]	[1]Wikipedia, Nicotine, http://en.wikipedia.org/wiki/Nicotine
HPropylene Glycol (anti-freeze)	Short term exposure causes eye, throat, and airway irritation. Long term inhalation exposure can result in children developing asthma [1, 2]. 90 percent of e-cigarette liquid [3].	[1] Wieslander, G; Norbäck, D; Lindgren, T. "*Experimental exposure to propylene glycol mist in aviation emergency training: acute ocular and respiratory effects.*" *Occupational and Environmental Medicine* 58:10 649-655, 2001. Choi, H; [2] Schmidbauer,N; Spengler,J; Bornehag, C., "*Sources of Propylene Glycol and Glycol Ethers in Air at Home,*" *International Journal of Environmental Research* and *Public Health* 7(12): 4213–4237, December 2010. [3] D. Palazzolo (2013), Electronic Cigarettes and Vaping: A New Challenge in Clinical Medicine and Public Health. A Literature Review, *Front Public Health*. 2013; 1: 56, http://www.ncbi.nlm.nih.gov/pmc/articles/PMC3859972/
Heavy metals such as tin, silver, nickel, cadmium and copper	Heavy metal poisoning can lead to cancer of many kinds. For instance, a biological dentist reported to me that root canal fillings can cause cancer in the body and metal fillings continually poison the body with every bite [1]. Known to be present and a risk but levels appear to be different for different products. Copper is found in some e-cigarette liquids [2]	Heavy metal contaminants are referred to above. Also see: American Heart Association policy statement on e-cigarettes and [1] G. Munro-Hall, "Toxic Dentistry Exposed", 2009, Browsebooks. [2] American Industrial Hygene Association (Oct 19 2014), White Paper: Electronic Cigarettes in the Indoor Environment, https://www.aiha.org/government-affairs/Documents/Electronc%20Cig%20Document_Final.pdf
Diacetyl	Is linked to the illness known as 'popcorn worker's lung.' [1]. In a separate study, Diacetyl was found in 39 of 51 e-cigarettes flavours tested [2]. The UK's National Health Service stunningly publicly downplayed this important finding: http://www.nhs.uk/news/2015/12December/Pages/Flavouring-found-in-e-cigarettes-linked-to-popcorn-lung.aspx. Just where do the NHS's interests really lie?	[1] METRO newspaper, 'E-cig refill linked to lung condition,' September 1st 2014, page 4. [2] J. Allen et al. (2015), "Flavoring Chemicals in E-Cigarettes: Diacetyl, 2,3-Pentanedione, and Acetoin in a Sample of 51 Products, Including Fruit-, Candy-, and Cocktail-Flavored E-Cigarettes", *Environmental Health Perspectives*, DOI:10.1289/ehp.1510185.

Flavourings (e.g. bubble gum): Aldehyde, vanillin, ethyl vanillin	Primary irritant of mucosal tissue of respiratory tract. Levels identified as a "toxicological concern". [1] Another study found two toxic chemicals, 2,3-Pentanedione, and Acetoin, in flavourings (as well as Diacetyl), in 47 of 51 e-cigarette tobacco flavourings [2].	[1] *Tobacco Control*, P. Tierney *et al.*, "Flavour chemicals in electronic cigarette fluids", published online 15 April 2015, http://tobaccocontrol.bmj.com/content/early/2015/03/27/tobaccocontrol-2014-052175.full [2] J. Allen et al. (2015), "Flavoring Chemicals in E-Cigarettes: Diacetyl, 2,3-Pentanedione, and Acetoin in a Sample of 51 Products, Including Fruit-, Candy-, and Cocktail-Flavored E-Cigarettes", *Environmental Health Perspectives*, DOI:10.1289/ehp.1510185.

Note that the table does not consider the amount of each toxin in terms of parts per million or billion except where it is reported. Are these levels comparable to those of tobacco? In some cases, yes; in some cases, more so; and in some cases a lot less so. Also, some of these ingredients may not be seen in tobacco cigarettes and many ingredients in tobacco cigarettes may not be seen in electronic cigarettes. So like-for-like comparisons are not entirely justified. What is the cumulative effect of all these toxins in the e-cigarette, not in terms of taking one-by-one but in terms of the synergistic effect? One combined with another? Or combined with 10 others? Or all combined together? These are unanswered questions – where are the studies? But the general scientific opinion thus far points to less toxins than tobacco and that they equate to less harm. But less toxins do not necessarily mean less harm; that which is currently found in e-cigarettes is very toxic even in tiny amounts. It's well known that the official safety limits of many toxins, poisons and carcinogens are too lenient; and sadly this is often to do with protecting the industry and its revenues rather than protecting people and the planet. For example, mercury from amalgams in our mouths is supposed to be safe but lower levels found in a factory would lead to its closure as unsafe. E-cigarettes are causing harm – they cannot fail to when you examine their ingredients. Will e-cigarettes help you quit smoking? It is safe to say, no, not according to the evidence. Over time, this may change but for now, the evidence is clear that e-cigarettes are not devices to quit smoking with.

Do e-cigarettes really help you quit tobacco?

E-cigarettes are *not* the answer to quitting tobacco; you will vape toxins rather than smoke them, swapping one poison for another. It may well be less poisonous to vape – let us hope so – but to still pour toxins into one's lungs and body is extremely dangerous. A paper published in *The Lancet*[58] found after a systematic review and meta-analysis of previously published studies that e-cigarettes actually _reduce_ the likelihood of smokers quitting by 28 per cent! One of the authors of this study, Professor Stanton Glantz, is quoted on CBS News as stating: "...the most dangerous thing about e-cigarettes is that they keep people smoking conventional cigarettes."[59]

In 2015 the U.S. Preventative Services Task Force stated:

"The USPSTF concludes that the current evidence is insufficient to recommend electronic nicotine delivery systems (ENDS) for tobacco cessation in adults, including pregnant women. The USPSTF recommends that clinicians direct patients who smoke tobacco to other cessation interventions with established effectiveness and safety."[60]

Despite this, in the UK at least, it could soon be possible to get e-cigarettes on prescription as tobacco smoking cessation devices. One-in-eight of the world's billion smokers smokes a tobacco cigarette made by British American Tobacco. BAT's e-cigarette, e-Voke, could be prescribed by the UK's National Health Service during 2016 because the UK's medicine regulator has approved a brand of e-cigarette for marketing as a smoking cessation device[61]. Isn't this contrary to the evidence? How can a national "health" service promote vaping? It is understood the need to get rid of tobacco cigarettes and actually that is easy at governmental levels: just ban them. But, as this is unlikely for some time whilst governments enjoy the tax revenues from tobacco, one then turns to the facts as reported here. On what evidence can governments give license to Big Tobacco to promote their products as healthy? All of the above indicates that it cannot be claimed that e-cigarettes help people quit and that it cannot be claimed that e-cigarettes are harmless. Yet, this is what the UK Government is effectively claiming, that there is negligible risk in e-cigarettes with regards to health and that they help in quitting smoking.

E-cigarettes do not burn so there is no tar, no carbon monoxide, which is deadly. Because of this, the UK Government's website, UK.gov, stated in August 2015 that e-cigarettes are 95% less harmful than smoking tobacco cigarettes[62]. So we can say that e-cigarettes in this respect are not as harmful as cigarettes but that's effectively ignoring all the carcinogens and toxins found in e-cigarettes that are reported in the scientific and medical literature. It is impossible to state that tobacco is 95% more harmful than e-cigarettes because there are no long-term studies of e-cigarette medical effects. But this is the implication from the UK Government. A smoker's health declines almost immediately from the first puff but the development of cancers and other serious illnesses to the point where treatment is required takes a significant number of years. The number of years we need to see the long-term health effects of electronic cigarettes will be the same before the conclusion the UK Government has prematurely stated may be drawn with any confidence.

Irrespective of the above, even if every tobacco smoker takes up e-cigarettes and quits tobacco smoking, then we will have to deal with all the long-term health effects of e-cigarettes that come from filling one's lungs with toxins and carcinogens, all of it dangerous and many people will die from cancers and other dreadful diseases, and live less than happy lives. Filling one's lungs with anything but clear air is not going to be healthy. Lungs are designed for air, not smoke or vapour full of poisons. The root cause of the problem is addiction to nicotine. Eliminate nicotine addiction and break the habit of vaping entirely. When people stop vaping, then they will stop filling their lungs and bodies with cancer and disease causing agents. There are some e-cigarettes that do not include nicotine – yet still this is not a healthy option because the vapour, as stated, still contains carcinogens and toxins, and disease will ensue.

Guidance on how to quit

The purpose of this book is to shed some light on the danger lurking in e-cigarettes and to present the evidence that people need to inform them to not take up vaping in the first place, nor tobacco for that matter. So the goal of this book was not to show how someone can quit. However, it is important to find a trusted source that can help people quit smoking and/or vaping. The most useful and practical information I have found, and I recommend most highly, can be located on the website of *The World Foundation for Natural Science*[63]. Though the content is aimed at smokers, the same applies for vaping because the key addictive drug in tobacco cigarettes is nicotine, the same addictive drug used in most e-cigarettes.

Concluding remarks

I want to re-iterate and be clear again: tobacco cigarettes are deadly and should immediately be banned permanently from the planet. So I am not saying people should continue to smoke. All I am saying is that the difference between tobacco and e-cigarettes is more blurred than we are led to believe by the marketers (including governments). E-cigarettes do have an advantage in that they do not smell like tobacco, a dreadful smell of death and decay. But, again to make a point, those pushing for a switch to electronic cigarettes as a healthy choice should be aware that e-cigarettes are not harmless. Far from it. The evidence shows the potential for much harm.

It has been shown that e-cigarettes contain a number of toxins, many of which are very poisonous and are rated as causing cancer. It is also clear that those who vape are addicted. They cannot give it up. Those youth who vape or have tried vaping are also much more likely to try tobacco cigarettes. We must be extremely vigilant in protecting the innocent children from these products. Their almost ubiquitous take up is more than alarming. The long-term consequences are not clear but they cannot be good because of the amount of poisons they contain. In twenty years will we see hospital beds full of vapers who have lung cancer or a cancer unique to the vapour they inhale? We can claim ignorance but that doesn't work anymore. You cannot claim to be intelligent yet accept that vaping is somehow entirely safe. People are smoking tobacco a fraction less than they used to and yet the poisons in tobacco have been made apparent for many years. It is time to take the same step with e-cigarettes in clearly pointing out their toxic ingredients, the effect these ingredients can have and strongly promote a better way than electronic cigarettes. For they are poisonous and addictive and they should be banned outright. Politicians who read this take note, the so-called victory over Big Tobacco and tobacco cigarettes through promotion of a switch to electronic cigarettes is indeed pyrrhic. The e-cigarette is not the solution. E-cigarettes are owned by Big Tobacco.

As of going to print, September 2016, it has been announced that there has been a drop in the number of tobacco smokers in England with one-in-five people smoking in 2012 to just under on-in-five in 2015, from 19.3 per cent in 2012 to 16.9 per cent in 2015.[64] One premise put forward for this significant fall is the take up of electronic cigarettes as an alternative. Indeed, the UK government states that three-in-five tobacco smokers use e-cigarettes and two-in-five have switched from tobacco to electronic cigarettes.[65]

It is wonderful that less people are smoking and may the number that still smoke tobacco products drop to zero. But I come back to the point of this book and that is to show there is significant evidence from credible sources that electronic cigarettes are harmful to health. E-cigarettes are another form of smoking. Perhaps less deadly than tobacco, but still containing deadly chemicals, toxins and heavy metals. So all we are seeing, if it is because of e-cigarette use that people are giving up tobacco (and this has not been proven, it remains conjecture and anecdotal), is a shift from one deadly poison – fast working, let's call it – to another poison – perhaps, but not yet proven, to be slower working. We may well see in twenty years – or less – a new wave of cancers, diseases and health problems caused by e-cigarettes.

So, I reiterate, the time has come to ban tobacco smoking outright and permanently, globally. The same should be done with electronic cigarettes. Electronic cigarette uptake does not mean someone has truly quit smoking; he or she is still smoking, but just by a different mechanism. And finally, in case we forget, the manufacturers of electronic cigarettes are Big Tobacco.

About the author

Karl Cox holds a PhD in Computer Science and currently works at the University of Brighton on the south coast of England within the College of Life, Health and Physical Sciences. He has published over 80 peer reviewed papers, articles and one text book. Dr Cox now focusses his research on ethics in how technologies are used to either benefit or harm mankind, the environment and the planet. Dr Cox firmly believes that if a product causes harm, even if it is really useful, an alternative product has to be found to perform the same function or the harm caused to be nullified and proven independently to be so. Dr Cox has spoken at many conferences and mostly recently was an invited speaker at The World Foundation for Natural Science 2015 Annual World Congress in Ulm, Germany, where he was invited to talk about the real harm that genetically modified organisms (GMO) and pesticides cause to the soils, the nature kingdom and people.

References

[1] A. Higham et al., (2016), "Electronic cigarette exposure triggers neutrophil inflammatory responses," *Journal of Respiratory Research* (17:56); http://respiratory-research.biomedcentral.com/articles/10.1186/s12931-016-0368-x

[2] p. 8 in: A. Higham et al., (2016), "Electronic cigarette exposure triggers neutrophil inflammatory responses," *Journal of Respiratory Research* (17:56); http://respiratory-research.biomedcentral.com/articles/10.1186/s12931-016-0368-x

[3] Philip J. Hilts (1996), *Smokescreen – the truth behind the tobacco industry cover-up*, Addison-Wesley, ISBN: 0201488361

[4] Barrington-Trimis, Jessica L. et al., "E-Cigarettes and Future Cigarette Use", *Pediatrics*, July 2016, VOLUME 138 / ISSUE 1, http://pediatrics.aappublications.org/content/138/1/e20160379

[5] Arrazola, R.A., Singh, T., Corey, C.G. et al., "Tobacco Use Among Middle and High School Students—United States, 2011-2014," *Morbidity and Mortality Weekly Report*, 64(14); 381-385, April 17, 2015, http://www.cdc.gov/mmwr/preview/mmwrhtml/mm6414a3.htm

[6] Martin McKee, Peter Allebeck, "Why the European Journal of Public Health will no longer publish tobacco industry-supported research", Volume 24, Issue 2, 1 April 2014, http://eurpub.oxfordjournals.org/content/24/2/182

[7] Fiona Godlee et al., "Journal policy on research funded by the tobacco industry", *BMJ* 2013;347:f5193

[8] *Evening Standard*, 18th February 2016, p.7, "E-cigs smoked by 2.2m in Britain".

[9] *Public Health England*, "Use of e-cigarettes in public places and workplaces: Advice to inform evidence-based policy making", July 2016, https://www.gov.uk/government/uploads/system/uploads/attachment_data/file/534586/PHE-advice-on-use-of-e-cigarettes-in-public-places-and-workplaces.PDF

[10] http://www.dailymail.co.uk/news/article-2517504/VIP-E-cigarette-advert-Im-Celebrity-provokes-parents-outrage.html

[11] http://www.theguardian.com/technology/2013/oct/28/british-american-tobacco-apologises-for-advertising-e-cigarette-in-kids-app

[12] http://www.dailymail.co.uk/news/article-2546554/Ex-Marlboro-Man-dies-smoking-related-respiratory-failure.html

[13] M. Andrade, G. Hastings, K. Angus (2013), "Promotion of electronic cigarettes: tobacco marketing reinvented?", *BMJ* 2013;347:f7473, http://www.bmj.com/content/347/bmj.f7473

[14] Stephen Pritchard (5th January 2014), "The reader's editor on… advertising e-cigarettes", *The Observer*, http://www.theguardian.com/theobserver/2014/jan/05/readers-editor-on-advertising-e-cigarettes

[15] L Bauld et al., (2014) "E-cigarette uptake and marketing", *Public Health England* PHE publications gateway number: 2014079

[16] The *METRO* newspaper (17 June 2014), "Smoked bacon? It's one of 7,700 e-cig flavours…", page 21.

[17] Callum Tennent (20 Feb 2014), "The Dutch have created an e-cigarette / Bluetooth speaker combo, and it is incredible," http://www.whatmobile.net/2014/02/20/watch-dutch-created-e-cigarettebluetooth-speaker-combo-incredible/

[18] de Andrade M, Hastings G, Angus K, Dixon D and Purves R (2013). "The Marketing of Electronic Cigarettes in the UK", *Cancer Research UK*: London http://www.cancerresearchuk.org/prod_consump/groups/cr_common/@nre/@pol/documents/generalcontent/cr_115991.pdf

[19] http://triblive.com/business/headlines/7334184-74/cigarettes-devices-fda#axzz3M36r2eoh

[20] *Action on Smoking and Health* (ASH), "Electronic cigarettes", November 2014, http://www.ash.org.uk/files/documents/ASH_715.pdf

[21] Herzog B, Gerberi J, Scott A. "Equity research: Vapor—Revolutionizing the tobacco industry." San Francisco, CA: *Wells Fargo Securities*, LLC, Equity Research Department; May 19 2014.

[22] *Wikipedia*, "Electronic Cigarette", http://en.wikipedia.org/wiki/Electronic_cigarette#History

[23] Charlotta Pisinger, "Why public health people are more worried than excited over e-cigarettes", *BMC Medicine*, 2014, 12:226 doi:10.1186/s12916-014-0226-y, http://www.biomedcentral.com/1741-7015/12/226

[24] *Dr Matthew Mintz's Blogspot* (June 1st 2009), http://drmintz.blogspot.co.uk/2009/06/more-on-electronic-cigarettes-or-e-cigs.html

[25] *National Institute on Drug Abuse*, "Is Nicotine Addictive?" July 2012, http://www.drugabuse.gov/publications/research-reports/tobacco/nicotine-addictive

[26] W. El-Delaimy et al., (2015), "E-Cigarette Use in the Past and Quitting Behavior in the Future: A Population-Based Study", *American Journal of Public Health*, Published online ahead of print April 16, 2015: e1–e7. doi:10.2105/AJPH.2014.302482 http://ajph.aphapublications.org/doi/abs/10.2105/AJPH.2014.302482

[27] *CBS Local News*, "Health: Changes May Soon Come For Electronic Cigarette Users In Philadelphia", 26th March 2014, http://philadelphia.cbslocal.com/2014/03/26/health-changes-may-soon-come-for-electronic-cigarette-users-in-philadelphia/

[28] Daniel Cressey (24 March 2014), "Electronic cigarettes 'don't aid quitting', study says," *Nature*, http://www.nature.com/news/electronic-cigarettes-don-t-aid-quitting-study-says-1.14918

[29] R. A. Grana, L. Popova, P. M. Ling (2014), "A Longitudinal Analysis of Electronic Cigarette Use and Smoking Cessation," *JAMA Intern Med.* Published online March 24, 2014, doi:10.1001/jamainternmed.2014.187

[30] *CDC Press Release*, "More than a quarter-million youth who had never smoked a cigarette used e-cigarettes in 2013", 25th August 2014, http://www.cdc.gov/media/releases/2014/p0825-e-cigarettes.html

[31] *CDC Press Release*, "E-cigarette use triples among middle and high school students in just one year", 16th April 2015, http://www.cdc.gov/media/releases/2015/p0416-e-cigarette-use.html

[32] *Welsh Government*, "Exposure to secondhand smoke in cars and e-cigarette use among 10-11 year old children in Wales", 3rd December 2014, http://wales.gov.uk/statistics-and-research/exposure-secondhand-smoke-cars-ecigarette-use-among-children/?lang=en

[33] *The Guardian* (9th June 2015) "Wales to introduce e-cigarette ban", http://www.theguardian.com/society/2015/jun/09/wales-e-cigarette-ban

[34] T. Wills et al. (2015), "Risk Factors for Exclusive E-Cigarette Use and Dual E-Cigarette Use and Tobacco Use in Adolescents", *Pediatrics*, 135, No. 1., http://pediatrics.aappublications.org/content/early/2014/12/09/peds.2014-0760

[35] *The Washington Post*, "Don't let Big Tobacco hook a new generation on nicotine with alluring ads for e-cigarettes", 16th April 2014, http://www.washingtonpost.com/local/dont-let-big-tobacco-hook-a-new-generation-on-nicotine-with-alluring-ads-for-e-cigarettes/2014/04/16/1acd08b2-c5a3-11e3-bf7a-be01a9b69cf1_story.html

[36] Senator Richard Durbin et al., (April 14th 2014), "Gateway to Addiction?" http://www.durbin.senate.gov/imo/media/doc/Report%20-%20E-Cigarettes%20with%20Cover.pdf

[37] WHO Framework Convention on Tobacco Control, "Draft summary of the second meeting of the fifth Bureau of the Conference of the Parties to the WHO FTCC Geneva", 13-14 November 2013 (COP/Bureau/5/2/ Draft SR 6

Dec 2013)
http://nicotinepolicy.net/documents/misc/WHObureausummary.pdf

[38] *The Telegraph*, "EU Vote on Electronic Cigarettes 'makes no sense'", 14th July 2013,
http://www.telegraph.co.uk/news/worldnews/europe/eu/10178573/EU-vote-on-electronic-cigarettes-makes-no-sense.html

[39] Jay M. Arena (1986), *Poisoning: Toxicology, Symptoms, Treatments*, Charles C Thomas Pub Ltd.

[40] *CDC Press Release*, "New CDC study finds dramatic increase in e-cigarette-related calls to poison centers", 3rd April 2014.
http://www.cdc.gov/media/releases/2014/p0403-e-cigarette-poison.html

[41] *The New York Times*, "Selling a Poison by the Barrel: Liquid Nicotine for E-Cigarettes", 23rd March 2014,
http://www.nytimes.com/2014/03/24/business/selling-a-poison-by-the-barrel-liquid-nicotine-for-e-cigarettes.html?_r=1

[42] *The Inquisitor*, "E-Cigarettes Tragedy: 'Vaping' Claims Life of Toddler", 13th December 2014
http://www.inquisitr.com/1677808/e-cigarettes-tragedy-vaping-claims-life-of-toddler/

[43] *BBC News*, as quoted in, "E-cigarettes to be stubbed out for under 18s", 26th January 2014, http://www.bbc.co.uk/news/uk-25900542,.

[44] http://www.fda.gov/NewsEvents/PublicHealthFocus/ucm172906.htm

[45] *The Daily Mail*, as quoted in: "E-cigarettes contain chemicals that make some 'as harmful as normal tobacco'", 26th August 2013,
http://www.dailymail.co.uk/health/article-2402108/E-cigarettes-harmful-cigarettes-cause-cancer-claims-study.html

[46] *Medical News Today*, "Electronic cigarettes can harm the lungs", 10th June 2013, http://www.medicalnewstoday.com/articles/249784.php

[47] *Reader's Digest*, as quoted in Hickling, "Burning Questions", June 2014, p.46.

[48] *Mercola.com* (28 May 2014) "Poisons from e-cigarettes and synthetic pot are surging", http://articles.mercola.com/sites/articles/archive/2014/05/28/e-cigarette-poisoning.aspx

[49] Americans for Nonsmokers' Rights (2014), as quoted in "Electronic (e-) cigarettes and Secondhand Aerosol", http://no-smoke.org/pdf/ecigarette-secondhand-aerosol.pdf

[50] T. Schripp et al., (2013) "Does e-cigarette consumption cause passive vaping?" *Indoor Air*, 23, 25-31.

[51] p.9. *Public Health England*, "Use of e-cigarettes in public places and workplaces: Advice to inform evidence-based policy making", July 2016 https://www.gov.uk/government/uploads/system/uploads/attachment_data/file/534586/PHE-advice-on-use-of-e-cigarettes-in-public-places-and-workplaces.PDF

[52] A. Bhatnagar et al. (2014), "Electronic Cigarettes: A Policy Statement From the American Heart Association", published online in *Circulation: Journal of the American Heart Association*, August 24th 2014. http://circ.ahajournals.org/content/early/2014/08/22/CIR.0000000000000107.citation

[53] *BBC News*, "WHO calls for indoor ban on e-cigarette use", 26 August 2014, http://www.bbc.co.uk/news/health-28937610

[54] *US Food and Drug Administration* Tobacco Products: "Vaporizers, E-Cigarettes, and other Electronic Nicotine Delivery Systems (ENDS)", (updated 30 August 2016) http://www.fda.gov/TobaccoProducts/Labeling/ProductsIngredientsComponents/ucm456610.htm

[55] *Evening Standard*, 11th February 2016, "E-cigarettes may be just as harmful to pregnant women as tobacco, scientists warn," http://www.standard.co.uk/news/health/ecigarettes-may-be-just-as-

harmful-for-pregnant-women-as-tobacco-scientists-warn-a3178651.html

[56] *AAAS* (12th Feb 2016), "Alternative Tobacco Products May Be Just As Dangerous As Cigarettes", http://www.aaas.org/news/alternative-tobacco-products-may-be-just-dangerous-cigarettes

[57] *The Guardian*, "Japan to investigate e-cigarette safety after formaldehyde findings", 28th November 2014, http://www.theguardian.com/society/2014/nov/28/japan-e-cigarette-safety

[58] S. Kalkhoran, S. Glantz (2016), "E-cigarettes and smoking cessation in real-world and clinical settings: a systematic review and meta-analysis", *The Lancet Respiratory Medicine*, 4 (2), pp.116-128.

[59] *CBS News* (January 14th 2016), "Study: E-cigarettes don't help smokers quit", http://www.cbsnews.com/news/e-cigarettes-dont-help-smokers-quit-study/

[60] *USPSFP*, September 2015, "Tobacco Smoking Cessation in Adults, Including Pregnant Women: Behavioral and Pharmacotherapy Interventions," http://www.uspreventiveservicestaskforce.org/Page/Document/UpdateSummaryFinal/tobacco-use-in-adults-and-pregnant-women-counseling-and-interventions1

[61] *BBC* (4th January 2016), "E-cigarette may become available on NHS", http://www.bbc.co.uk/news/health-35221292

[62] *UK Government* (2015), "Press release: E-cigarettes around 95% less harmful than tobacco estimates landmark review", https://www.gov.uk/government/news/e-cigarettes-around-95-less-harmful-than-tobacco-estimates-landmark-review

[63] *The World Foundation for Natural Science*, "How to quit smoking", http://www.naturalscience.org/topics/health/smoking/how-to-quit-smoking/

[64] *BBC News*, "Smoking rates in England fall to lowest on record", 20 September 2016, http://www.bbc.co.uk/news/health-37406105

[65] *Public Health England*, "Health matters: smoking and quitting in England", 15 September 2015, https://www.gov.uk/government/publications/health-matters-smoking-and-quitting-in-england/smoking-and-quitting-in-england

www.ingramcontent.com/pod-product-compliance
Lightning Source LLC
Chambersburg PA
CBHW070242290526
45789CB00004B/1724